I t feels great to be he[...]
to jump and sho[...],
run with your friends
and feel the wind in your face.

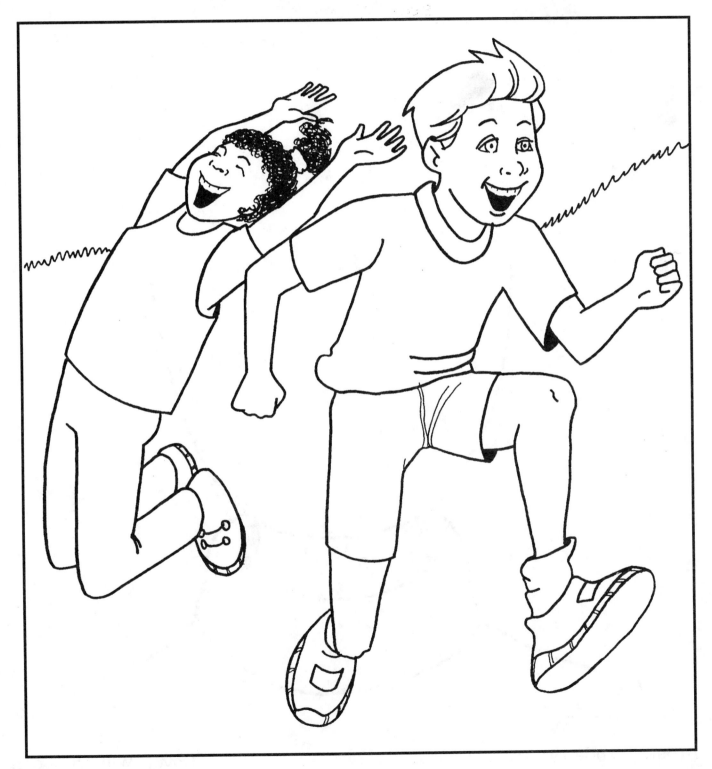

<u>YOUR NAME</u>

1

Draw a face showing how you feel today.

Hi! I'm Elfo, your guide.

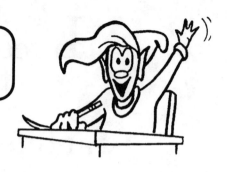

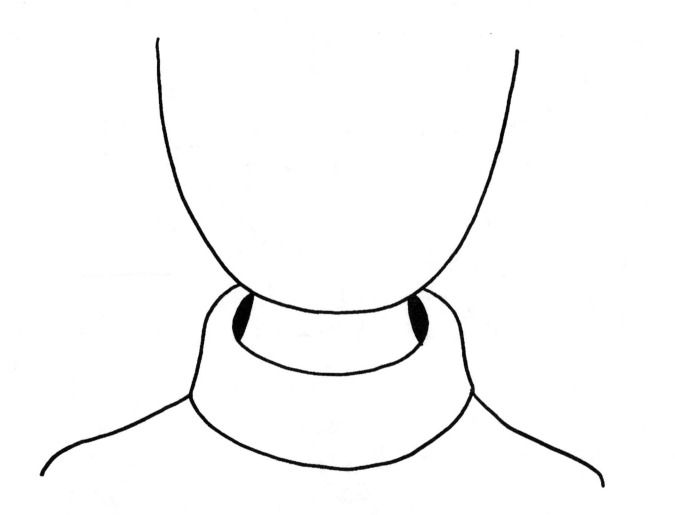

Artist: Brenda Brown

Cover: Wilfred Spoon

Copyright © 1995 by James B. Boulden
Printed in the USA
BOULDEN PUBLISHING, P.O. Box 1186, Weaverville, CA 96093

You want your friends and family
to be as healthy as you are.
But this is not always possible.

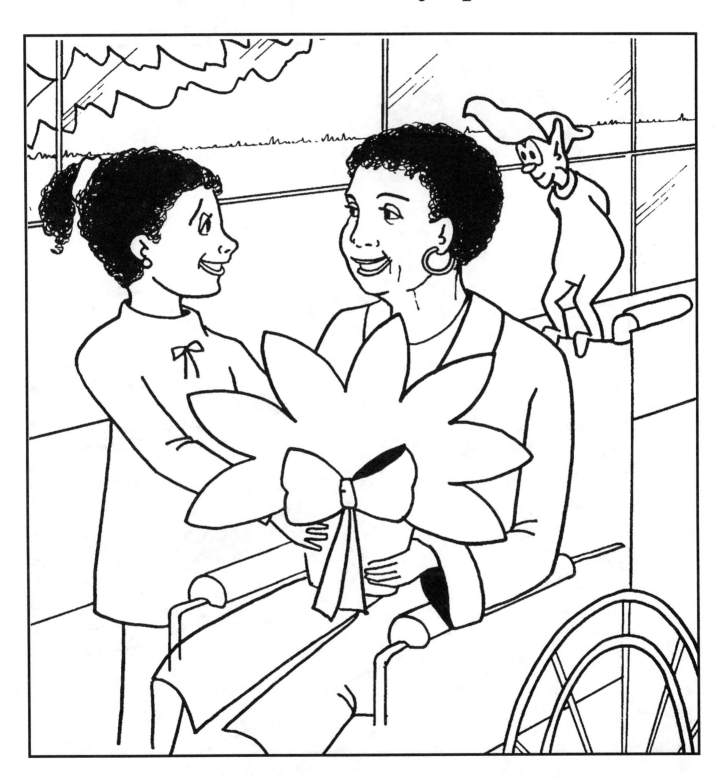

Who do you know that is very sick ?

All of us get sick or hurt at some time in our life. Usually, we feel fine again after a few days.

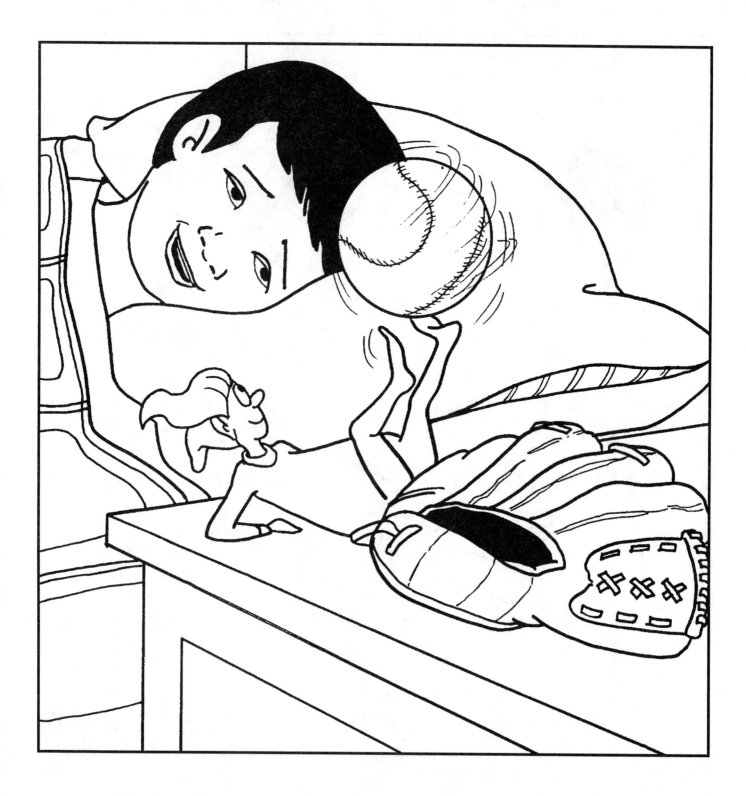

Tell about a time when you were sick.

Other times it is hard for people to get well. Doctors and nurses will do everything they can to help. Still your special person may stay sick for a long time.

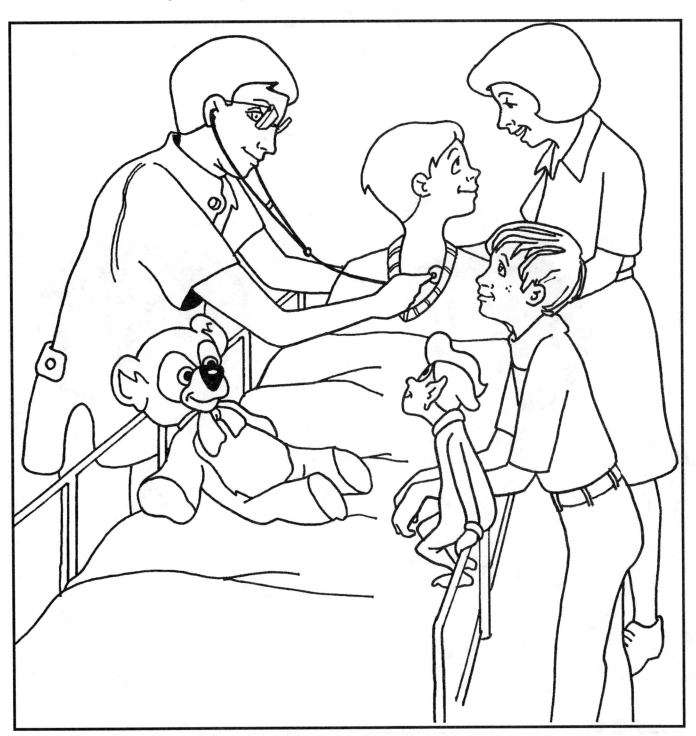

What have you been told is the cause of your special person being sick?

Your special person may have tubes
to feed them and machines to
watch over them.

Sometimes the machines make funny
noises like whirr whirr and beep beep.

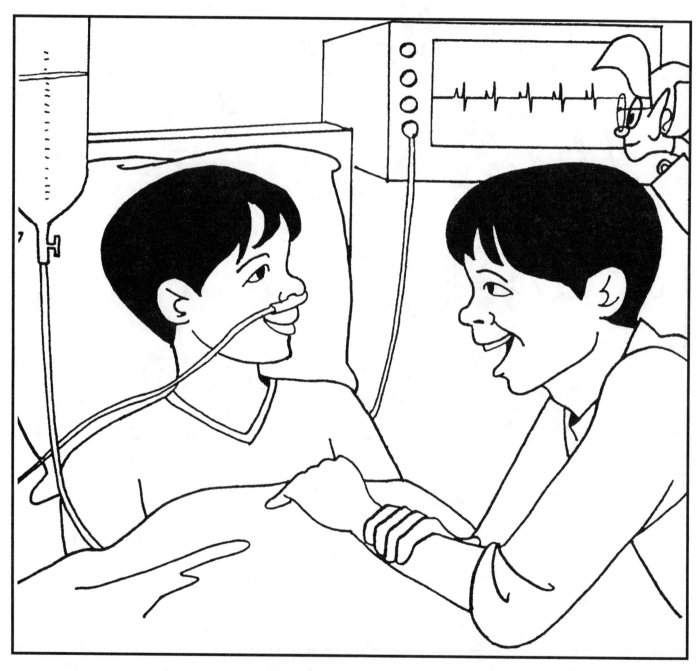

*How do you feel when you visit
your special person?*

Sick people often lose weight so that they look thin and different. They may take medicines that make their hair fall out. Then they may wear a wig.

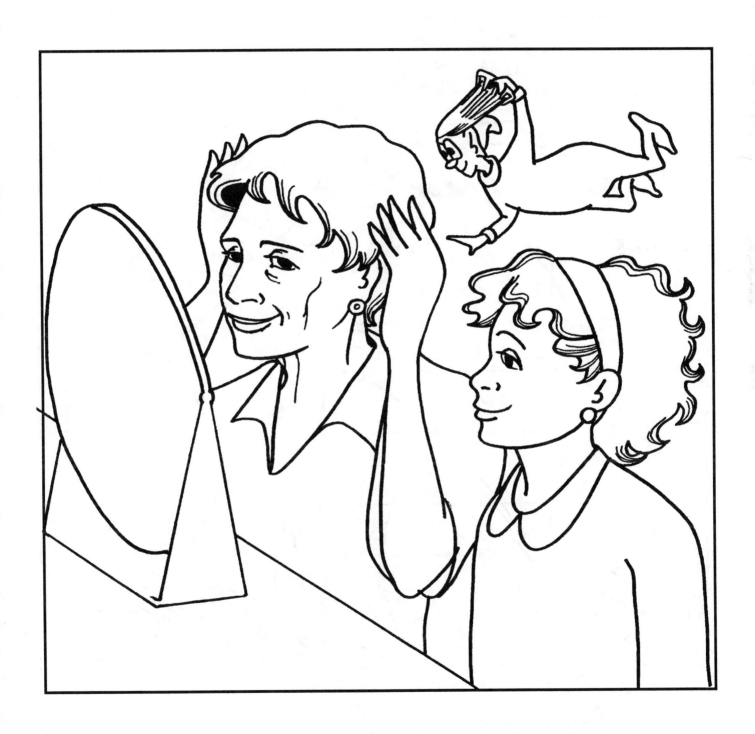

How does your special person look?

It may upset you to visit or be with your special person who is very sick.
You can let them know that you care for them because of who they are and not how they look.

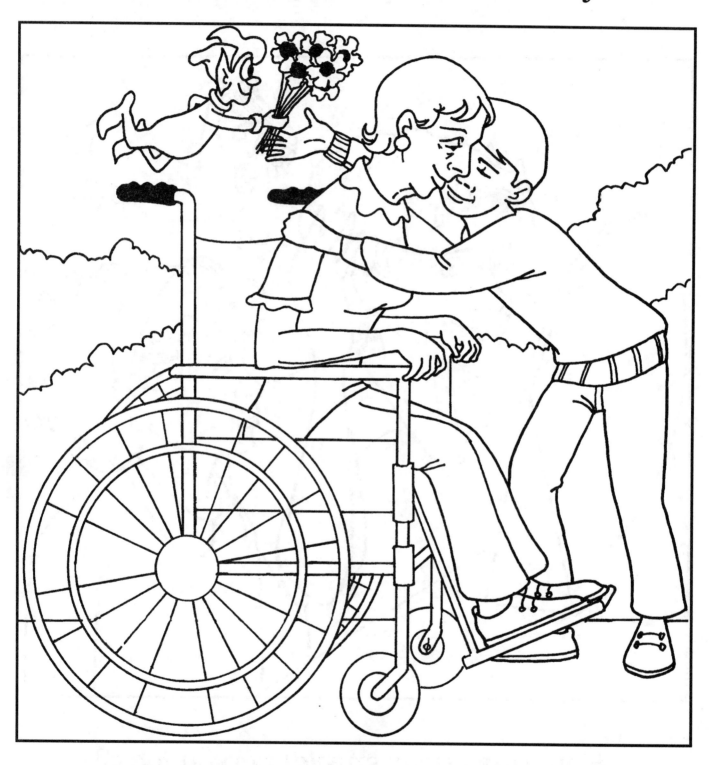

What can you say to a very sick person?

Your special person may take strong
medicines that make them sleep a lot.
Don't worry. The sleep is good for them.

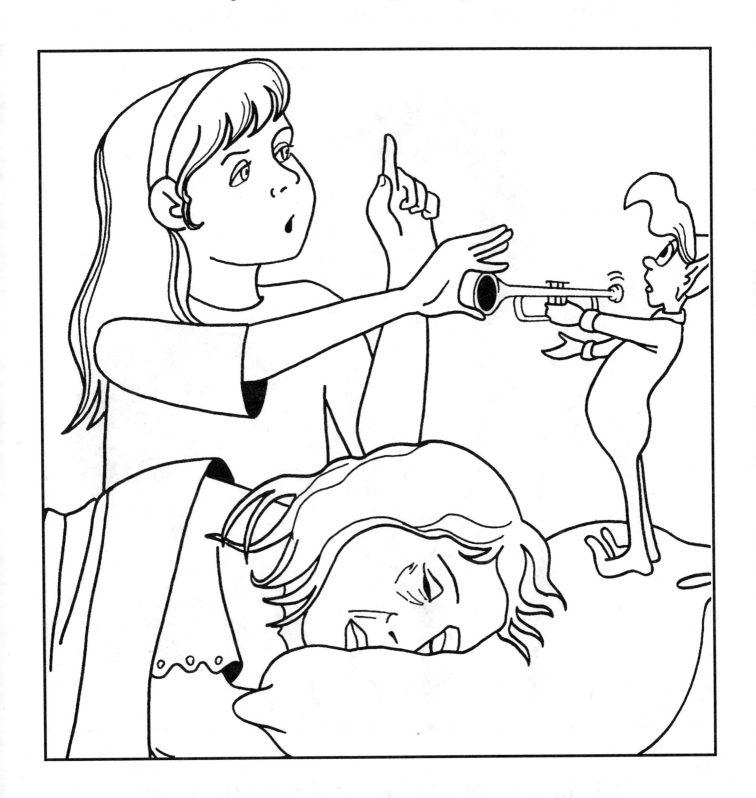

What can you do to help the sick person rest?

You may have many different feelings when someone close to you becomes sick. You may feel sad that your person is hurting. You may worry that you may also get sick.

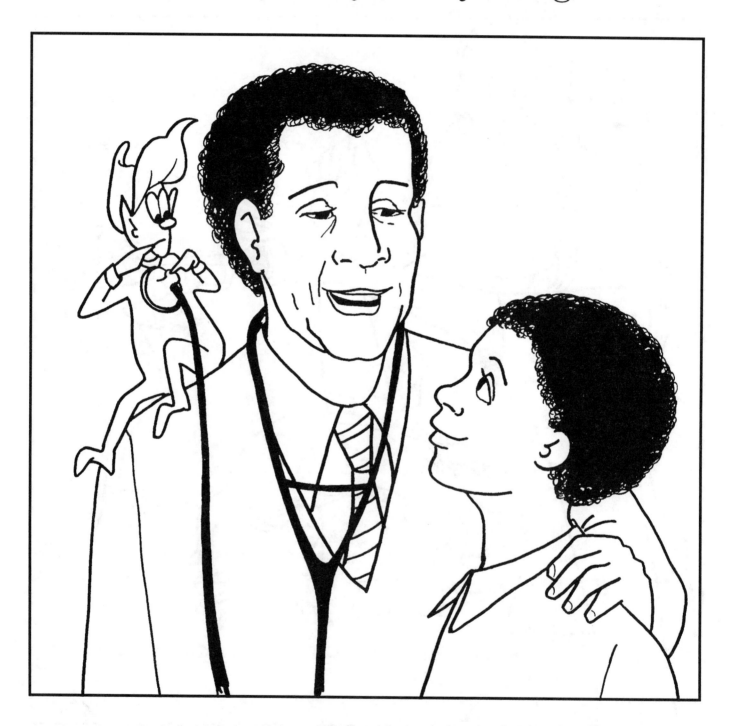

Who do you know that can answer your questions about the illness?

You may feel angry at the sick person for getting sick. It may seem that your family has forgotten you. This is not true.

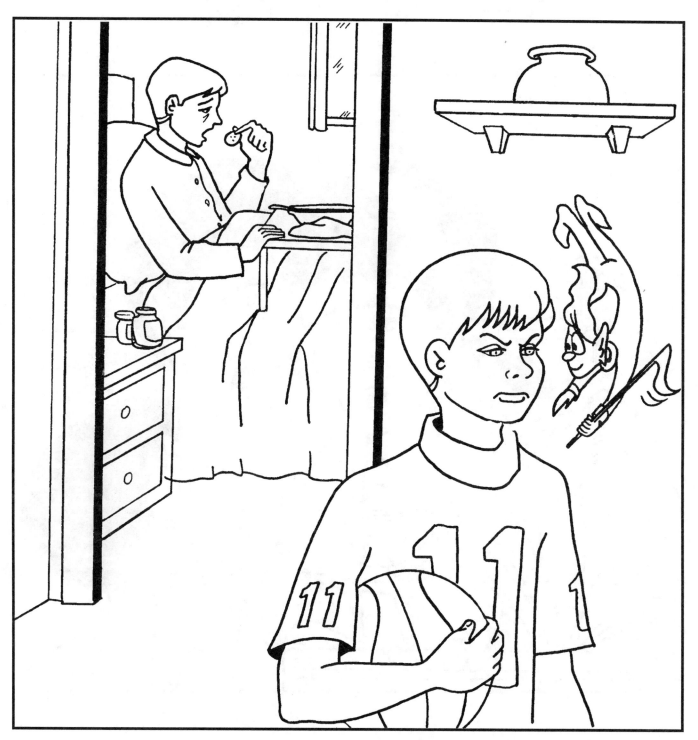

What can you do to help yourself feel better when you are angry and upset?

It is okay for you to feel the way you feel.

You may see grown-ups cry and
you can do that too.

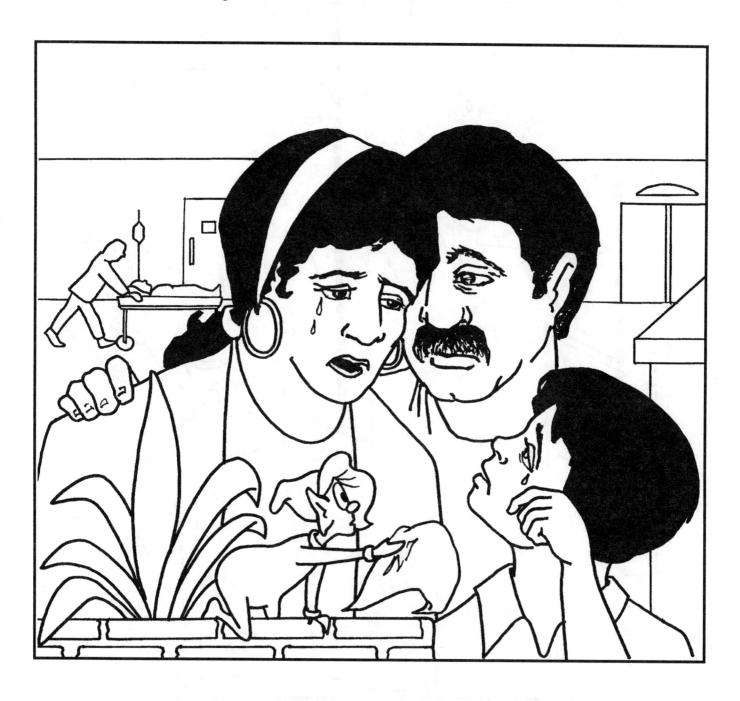

How would you feel about
other people seeing you cry?

You may be afraid that the sick person may never get well.

You can be sure that if that happens, there will be someone to take care of you. You are not alone.

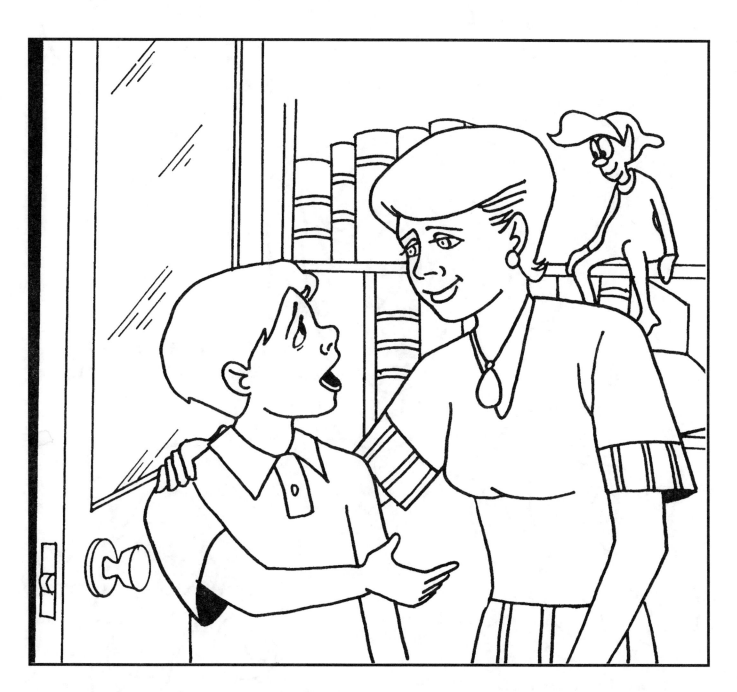

Who can you talk to about your feelings?

Color the faces that show how you feel about the sickness of your special person.

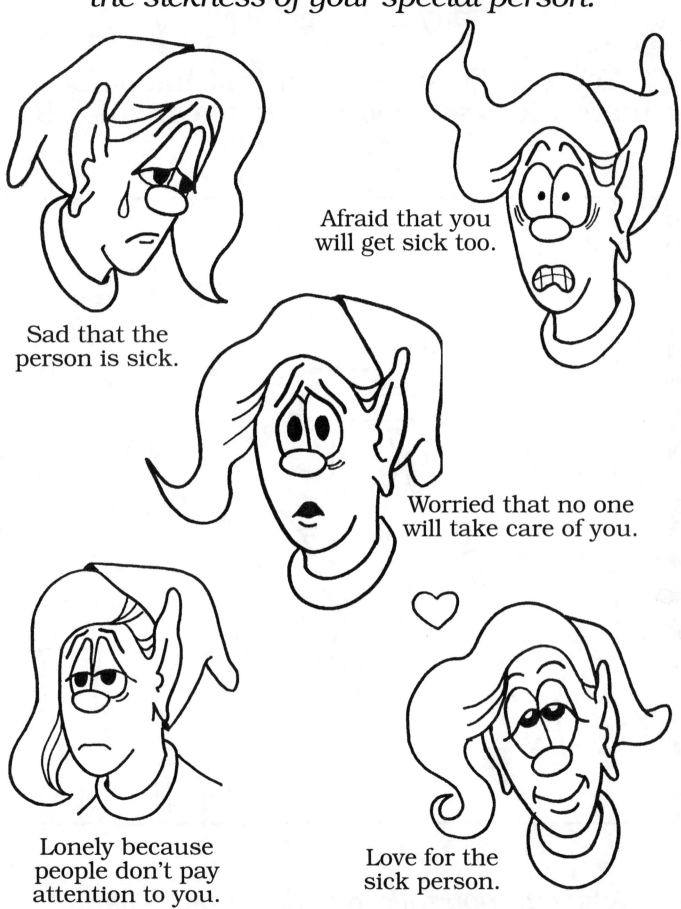

Sad that the person is sick.

Afraid that you will get sick too.

Worried that no one will take care of you.

Lonely because people don't pay attention to you.

Love for the sick person.

14

Things you can do when someone you care about is very sick.

Sit with the sick person.
It is not necessary to talk unless you feel like it.

Touch the sick person.
Let them know that they are not alone and that you care.

Be understanding when adults are cranky.
Sickness is hard on everyone.

Don't be afraid to show your feelings.
Tears can wash away the hurt.

Learn to do some things for yourself.
Adults may be busy taking care of the sick person.

Help take care of the house.
Pick up your toys and keep your room clean.

Play quietly when you are inside.
The sick person may be resting.

Don't touch any medicines or bandages.
They can make you very sick.

Talk to someone you trust about your feelings.
It is okay to feel however you feel.

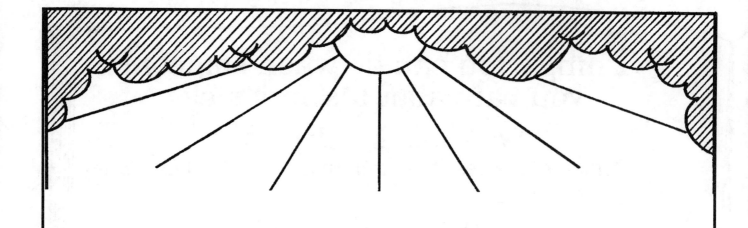

Draw a picture to help cheer your sick person.

CONTRIBUTING EDITORS TO THIS PUBLICATION
Lorie Armijo, Sharon Baker-Parks, Debbie DiBauda,
Jo Eekhoff, Judith German, Sue Murtaugh, Beverly Norfleet, Stacy Orloff, Carol Patacca, M. J. Seals,
Cherri Stefanic, Alice Teagarden, Judy Welsh, Lynn Wolfe

ADDITIONAL RESOURCES FOR CHILDREN IN DISTRESS
Phone (800) 238-8433 for free brochure.
Boulden Publishing; P.O.Box 1186, Weaverville, CA 96093